DUST

A BOOK FOR BROKEN PEOPLE

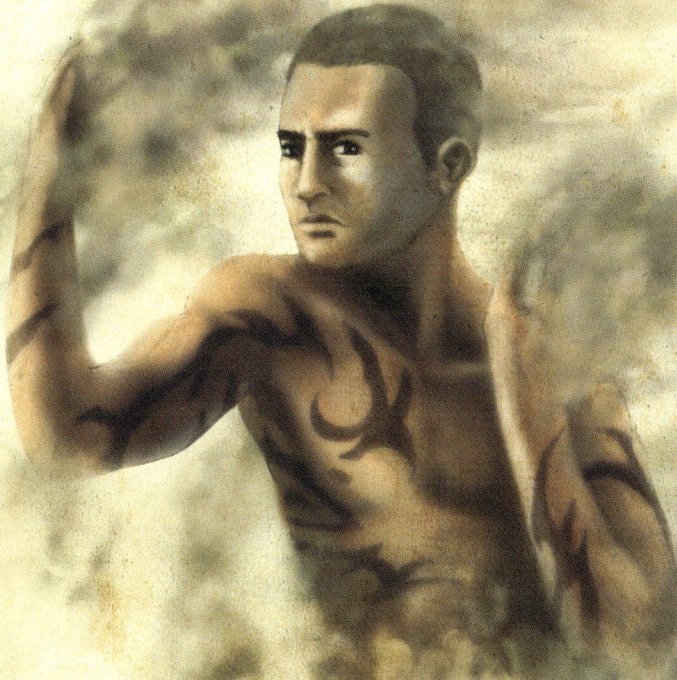

SHERRI GOUGH

Outskirts Press, Inc.
Denver, Colorado

This book is dedicated to the addict with no place to turn, the depressed with nothing to hope for, the lonely with no one to love them, the outcast, the misfit, the unworthy, the people who have made a mess of their lives and hurt other people while doing it, the sinner, the scarred, and the broken.

You are loved.

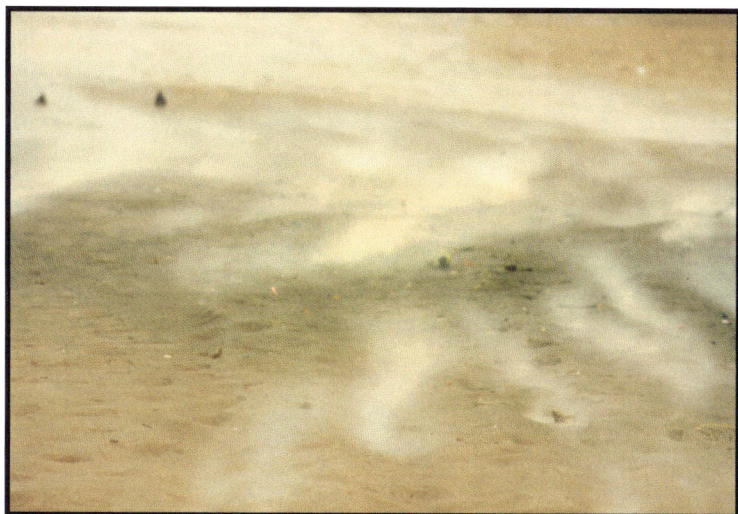

I am nothing. I am no one. I am just a bunch of dust put together, and nobody likes dust. Dust can't do anything, say anything, think anything. I'm just here, trying to hide from the nothingness that I am. Worthless. What can I do anyway?

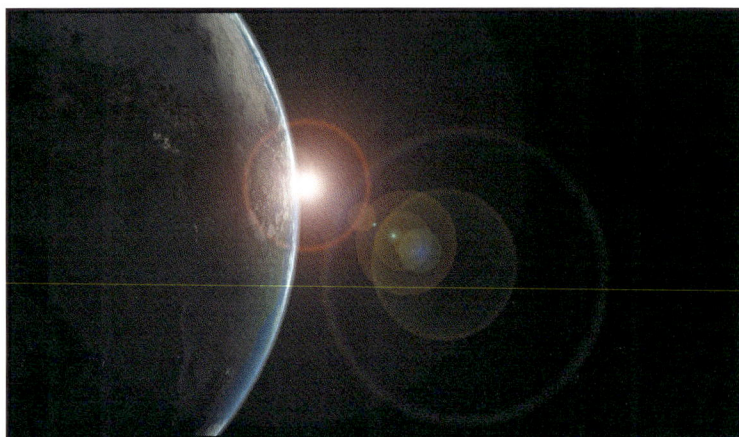

If I went away, the world would continue to go on just as it always has. And this ball of dust would be gone. No big deal. Just one ball of dust among so many. No one would even notice. There are so many balls of dust just floating around this world.

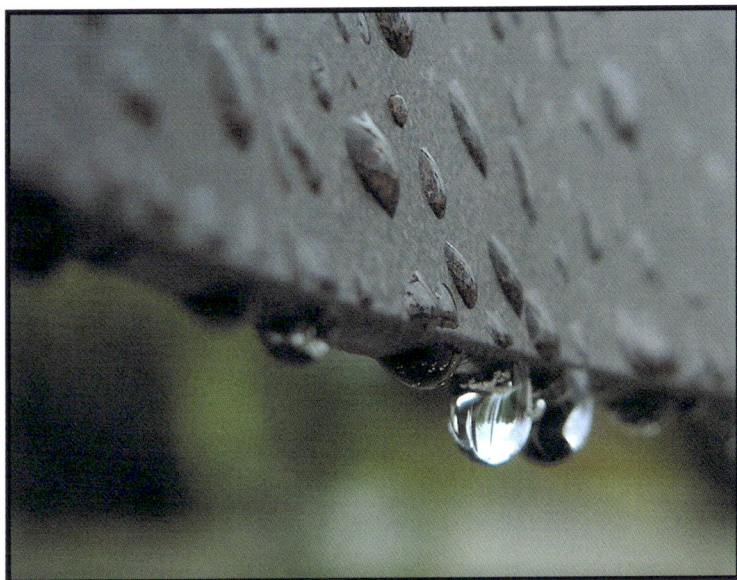

Yeah, I know God made me and everything, but as I sit here in agony he is silent. Would he even care if I disappeared? Would he do anything? Cry? Make a thunderstorm to show his sadness and grief? Probably not. The earth would just keep on turning.

Why did God even make the earth? Was it just an art project, so he could have something to do? Just like he made all the other planets? I wonder if God sits up there and makes a new planet every day just for fun. There are so many trillions of planets and stars and stuff. Maybe he tries to outdo himself every time just for a challenge and make a better planet than the day before.

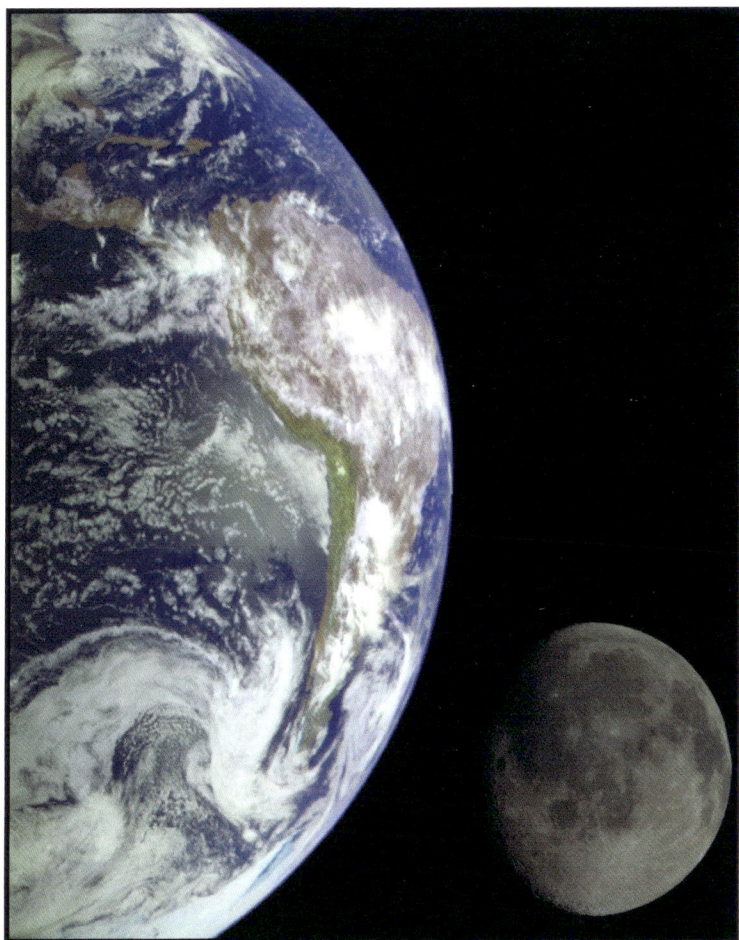

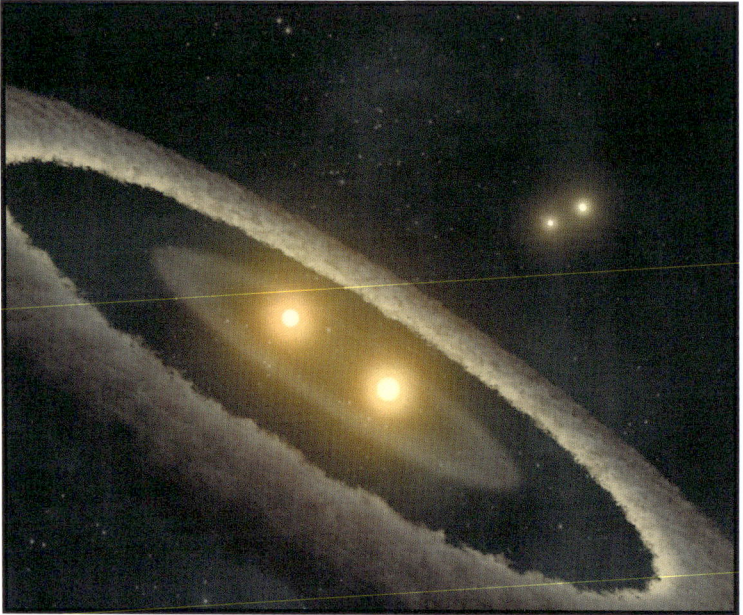

And what about stars? I think that would be cool. Creating something so huge that burns for millions of years and never stops. God must have fun up there.

∽ 6 ∾

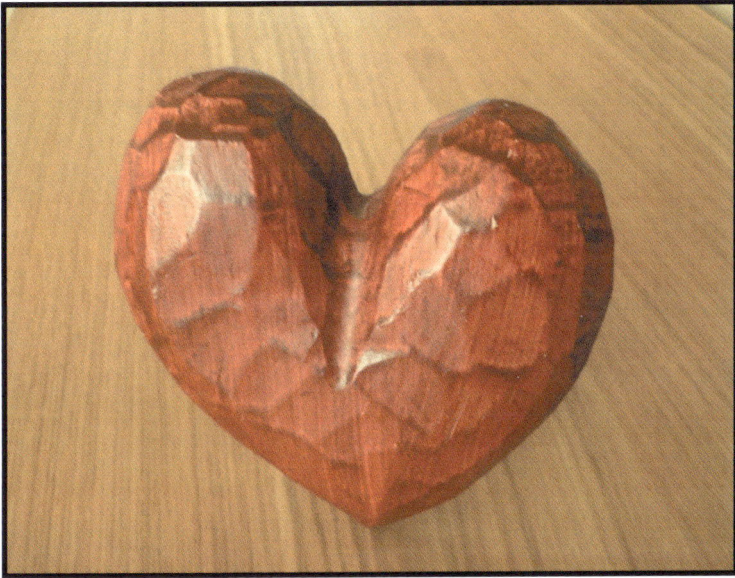

So if God is so huge, why did he make me? Why bother? Why did he put all the cells together to make my eyes? Or make all my veins so that blood could reach every single cell in my body? Or create my heart that keeps beating over and over without stopping. Kinda like that star up there that keeps on burning.

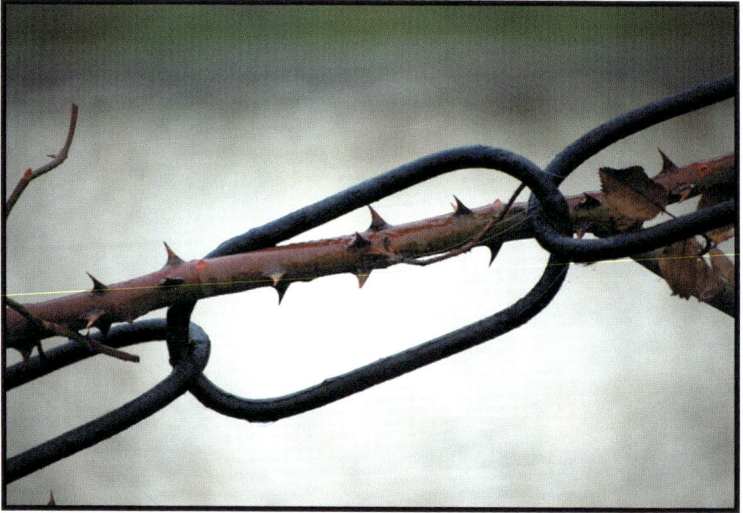

And what about feelings anyway?
Why did he give me those? They
just make me realize how bad life
is. I don't get it. If God is love
then why didn't he just make us
feel love and not pain.

෴ 8 ෴

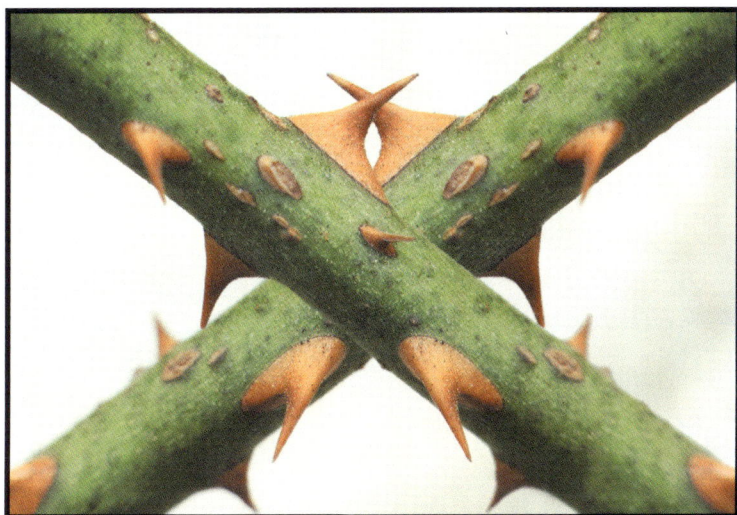

I wonder if he feels what I feel,
if he hurts because I hurt, if he
feels pain because of my pain, pain
because of love. And if he does,
then why is he so silent?

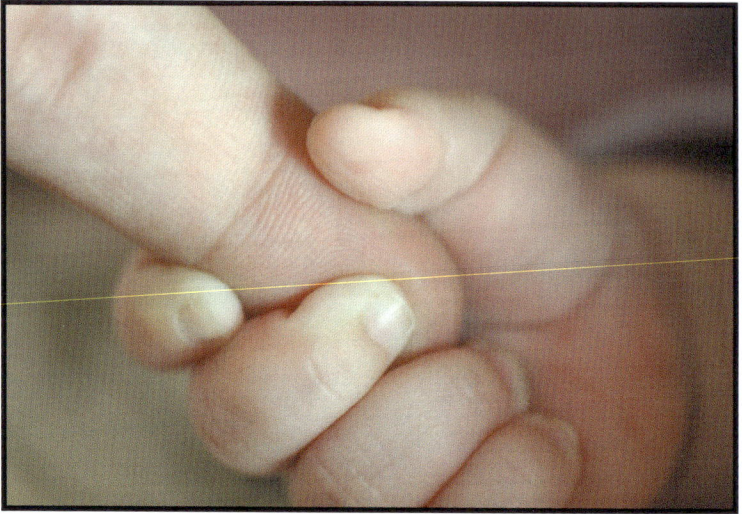

God must have loved me at some point in my life though because he went through all the trouble of creating me. And he didn't just wad up a ball of clay and say "there's my creation." Everything is really complex.

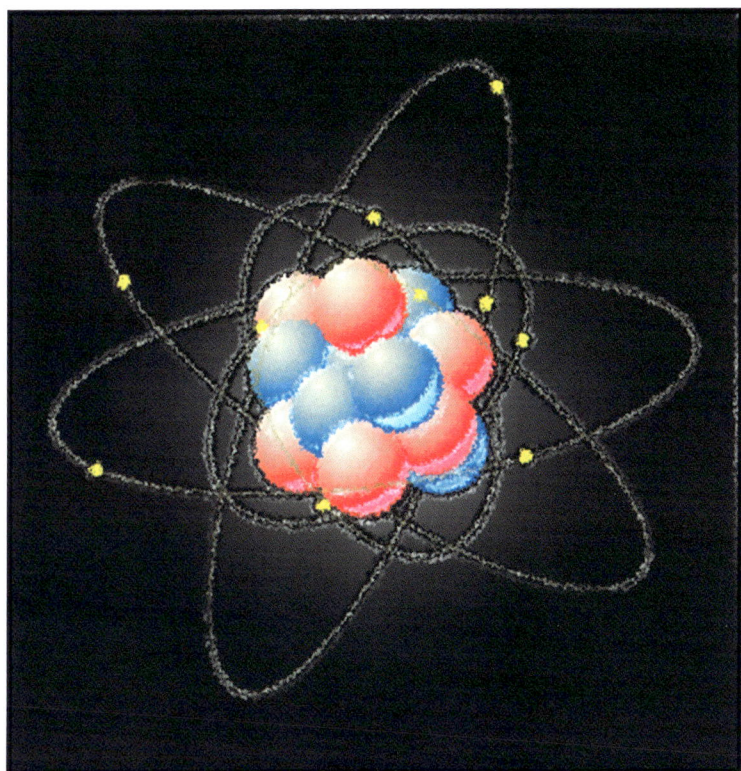

Those tiny little cells in my body are small, but they are bigger than all that scientific stuff that's really really small. Atoms, protons, neutrons, electrons. All of them are working without me knowing it or feeling it. I'm lying here and all of those tiny little things are still spinning and doing whatever they do.

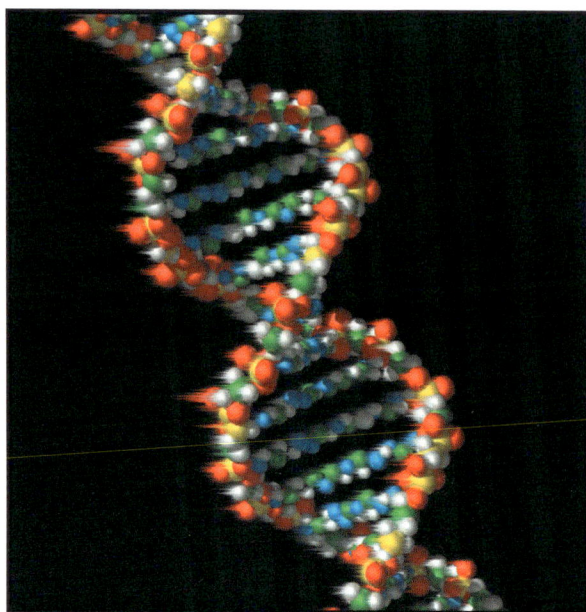

And of course my DNA...that's about the smallest thing I think. My DNA. MY DNA. Mine. Why would he make something to set me apart from everyone else? If I disappeared, my DNA would be gone from this world. Not like anyone would care. But it does make me different than everyone else I guess. A different ball of dust than all the rest. A ball of dust floating around that has something that no one else has...my own DNA. Yeah, cool. But who cares?

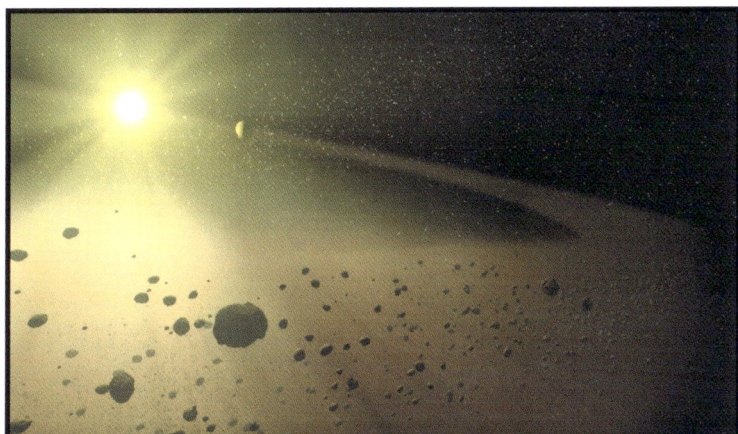

Still, why would God do that? Why would he make stars so big and wonderful and powerful and then make my DNA that is so small and seems so helpless right now? And it's not doing any good because I'm just lying here doing nothing. God made this incredible stuff and put it inside me and now I'm just lying here. Why did he even bother? Stars don't have DNA. Why didn't he give those really cool exploding things DNA instead of me?

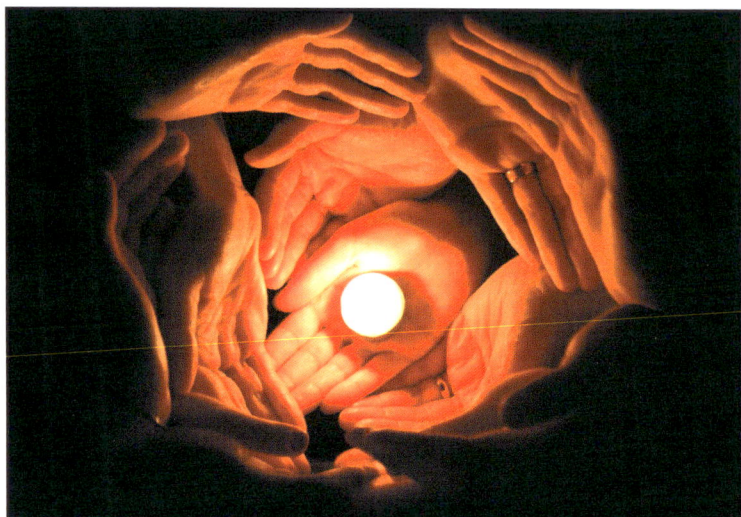

And why does he seem to send
people to me to care? Because a lot
of people, those other balls of dust
floating around, seem to care about
me, or at least they say they do.
Maybe God isn't so silent after all.
They are just DNA dust balls too.
And so I guess every one of them
is different, just like I'm different.

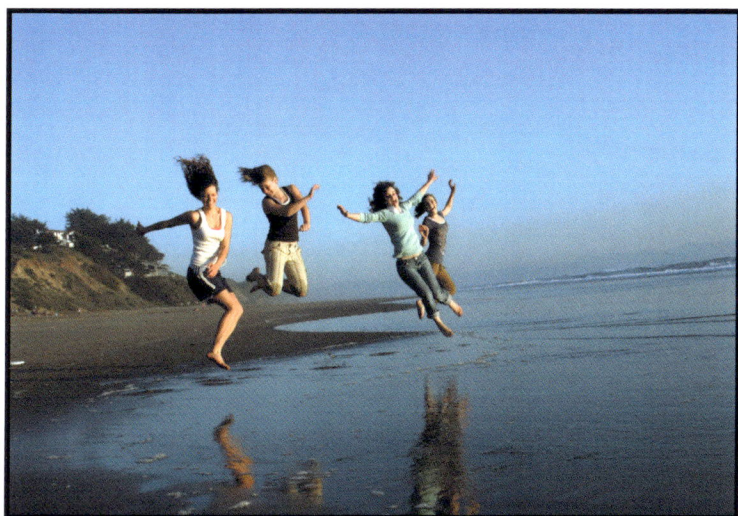

God made me. He shaped my body and made me different and gives me thoughts that no one else thinks, and relationships that no one else has. I guess everyone has friends, even some of the same friends as me, but not exactly the same relationships that I have.

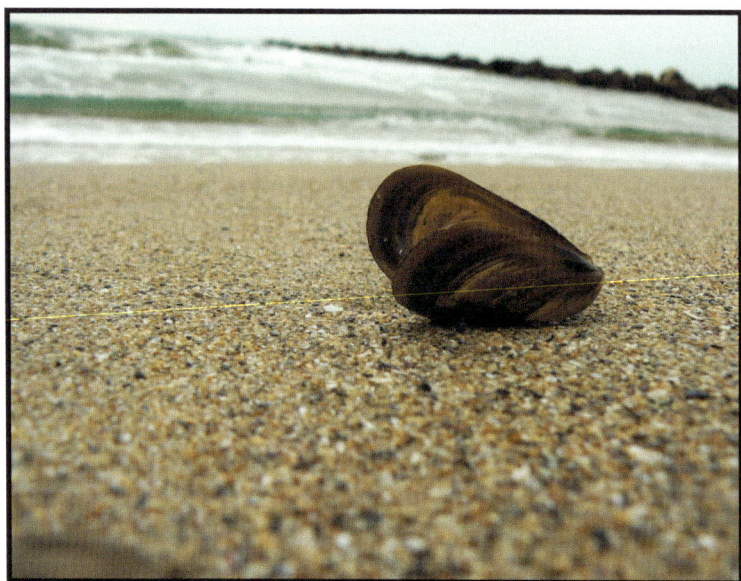

I know my friends care about me, but sometimes it still feels like I'm so alone. Alone. By myself in this world. Set apart. Created by God to be different. Alone. Only one person. One pile of dust in the middle of so many.

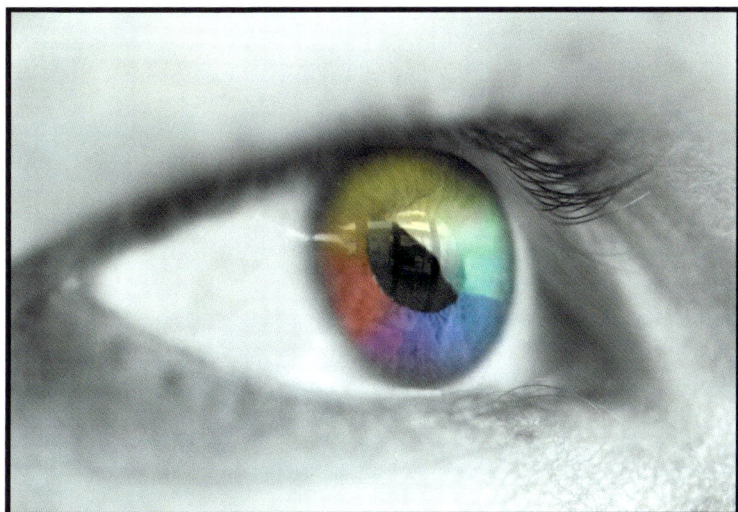

Lots of people do lots of things on this earth, even if they are just dust balls too, but none of them can be me. No one can think my thoughts, feel my feelings, see through my eyes or experience my blood running through my veins. No one. No one but me.

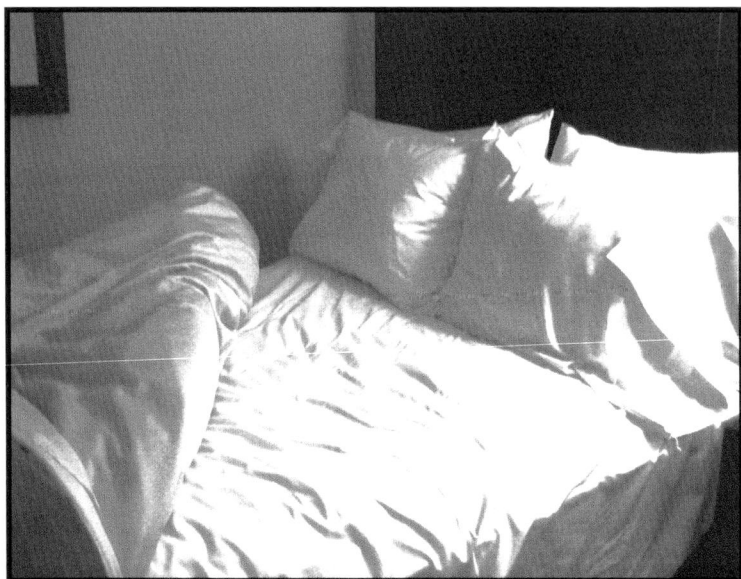

So maybe I am doing something after all just lying here. I'm existing. And I'm the only one who can exist for myself. But what can I do? My life is really screwed up. I can't help anybody. I can't even find the will to get out of bed in the morning.

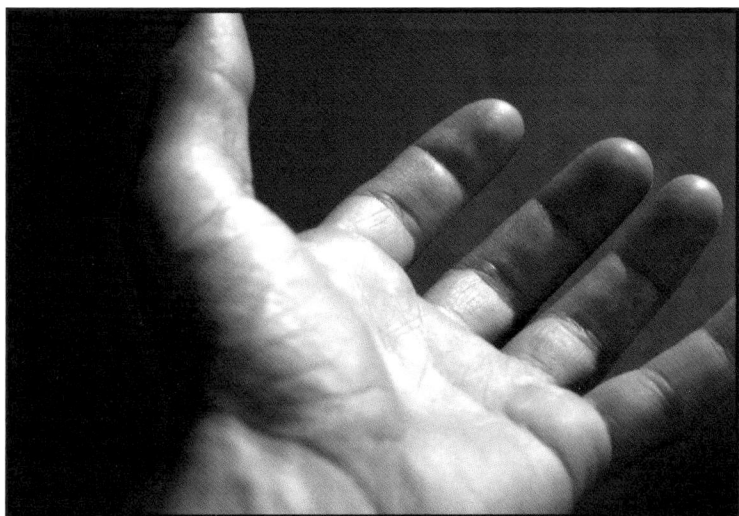

But I can exist. After all, God went through so much trouble to get everything right, give me my own DNA, and even, at some moment, reached his hand down and started my heart beating. If he would do that for me, then I can exist for him I suppose.

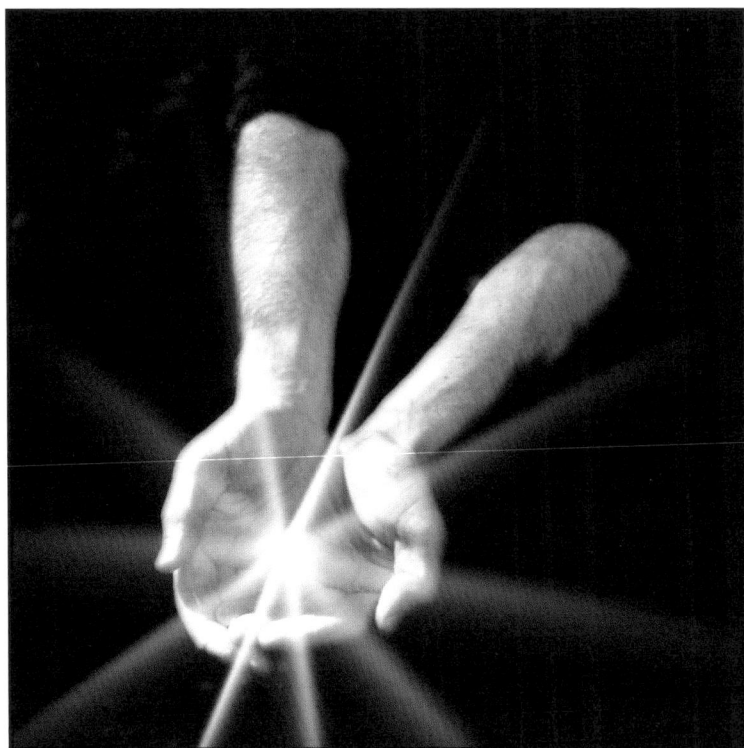

So what now? I don't have the will to do anything. I just want to disappear. Do you think it's possible for God to reach his hands down here to hold me? Cause if he brought them down here to start my heart beating, then it's possible for him to do it now, isn't it?

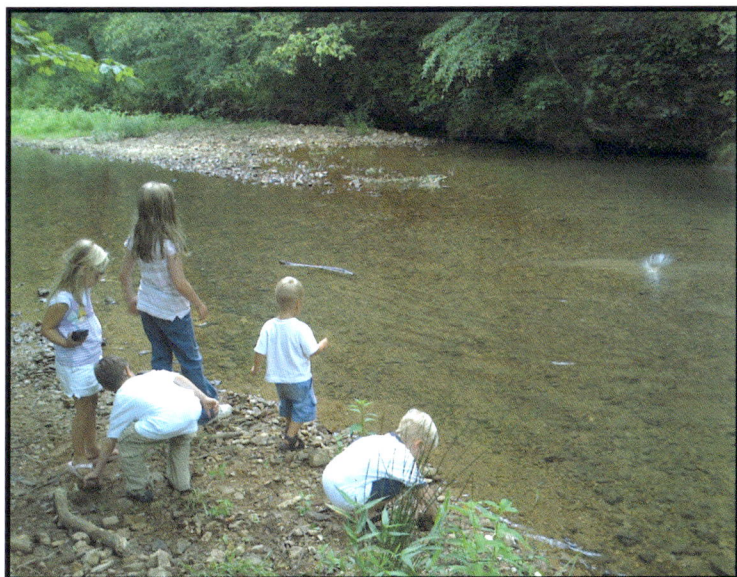

Even in my pain, in the back of my mind are memories. Good and bad memories, but some of them are good. And I remember all of the people I have come into contact with in some way and the things I've done in the past.

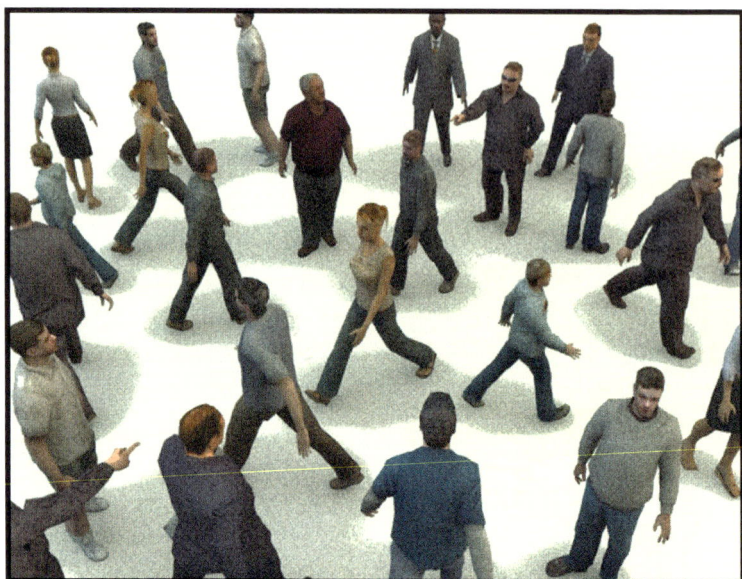

How many people know me? My family of course, even though sometimes it doesn't seem like they care. Everyone I've talked to. Everyone I've met in my life. The guy who owns the pizza store. The girl at the bank. The kids that live next door. The grocery clerk who bags my groceries. Everyone at every place I've been in my life. How many people, if I disappeared, would say, "Hey, I know him, he... (did whatever)..."

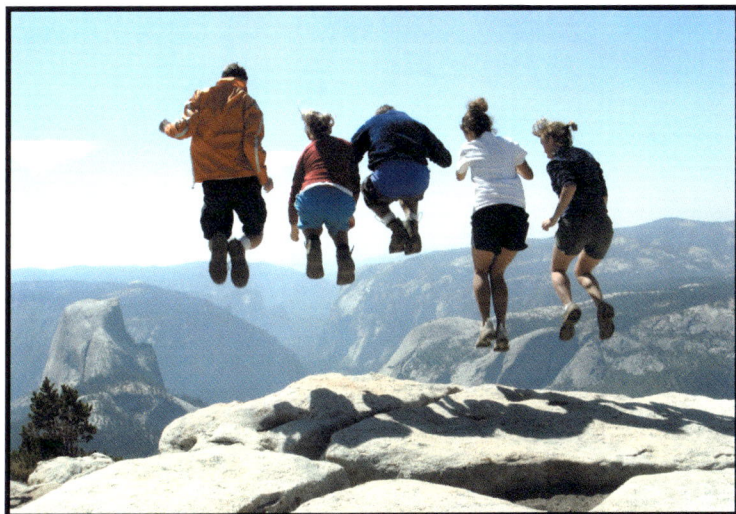

How many memories have I made here on this earth? How many people's lives have I touched, unaware that I was touching them, just by coming into contact with them at some point in my, and their, existence?

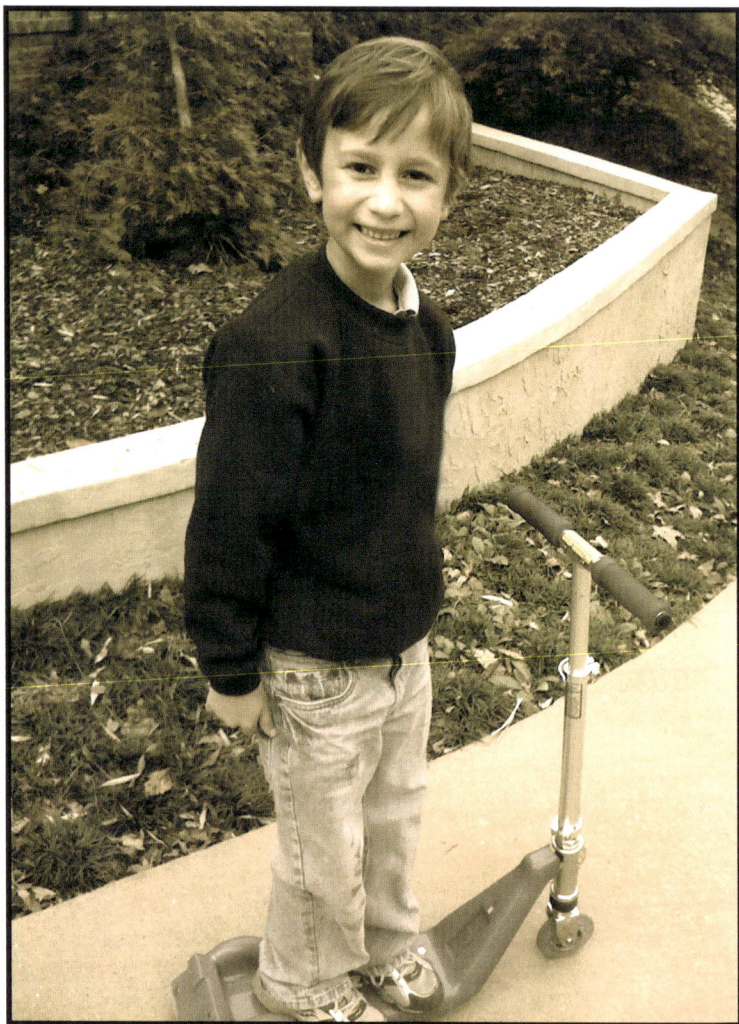

If I disappeared, who would I be letting down? The little boy down the street? What would he think? Everyone in my town? What would they think? The people who are closest to me? What would they think? God? What would he think? God. The one who put all the pieces together that make me ME and made sure that they all work. It's kinda like magic, really, how I'm created with such little pieces that all fit together. Pieces I can't even see.

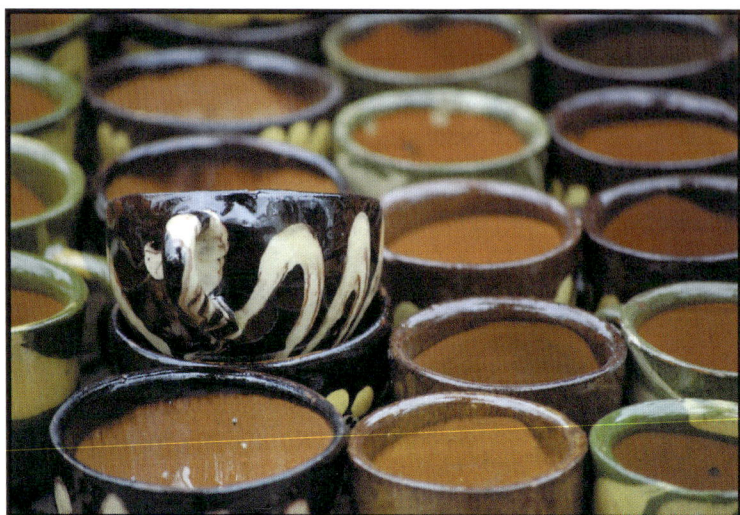

I am a miracle. It's a miracle that
everything put together, all of
this "dust," makes me who I am.
But it's special dust because no
one else has it. No one else is or
can ever have what I have, or can
ever be what I can be. No one can
ever affect the people that I can
affect in the way that I can. No
one. Not Bill Gates or Brad Pitt or
the President. They can do a lot
of things and lots of people like
them, but they can't be me. Ever.

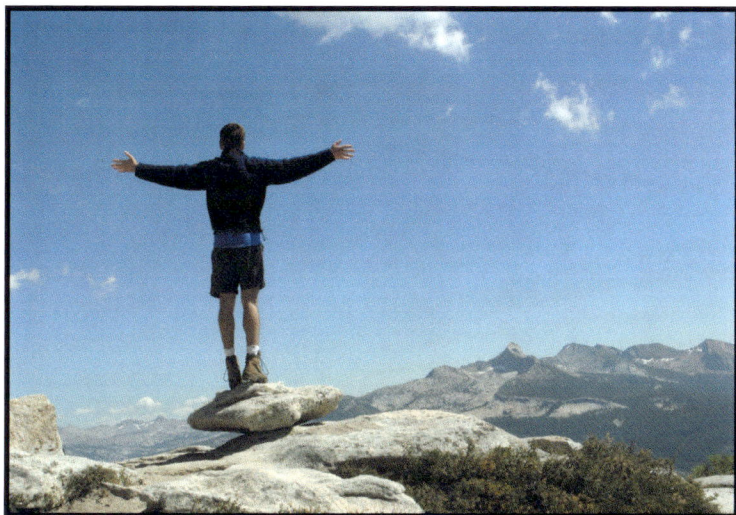

They can never feel the wind on my face, or smile the way that I smile, or think my thoughts. Ever. They can never affect the little boy down the street the way I can. They can affect him, but not exactly the same way that I can. Ever. Because they're not me, and each of the relationships that I have is special.

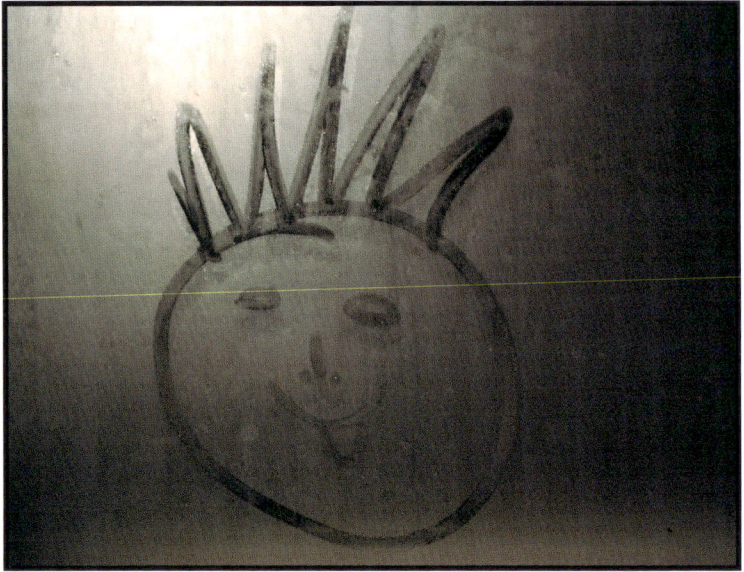

They can never feel my heart beat
inside of me, the heart that God
reached down to start, and they
can never feel my joy or my pain.
Only I can do that stuff. Only me.

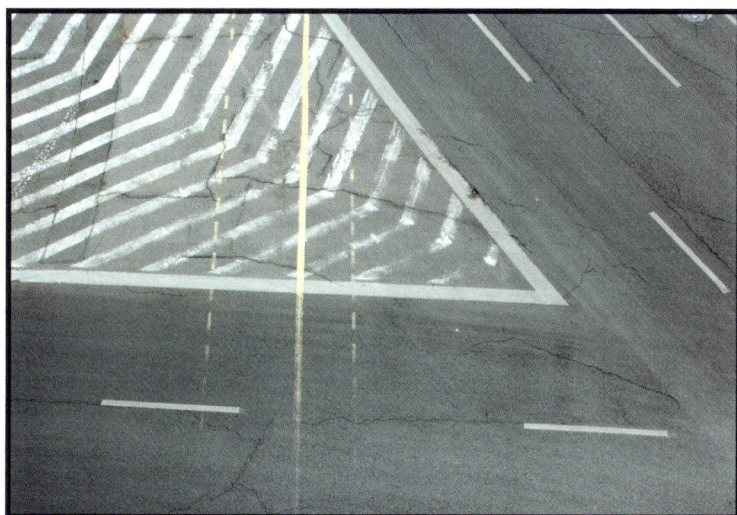

And only I can decide to keep going by myself or turn my life over to God. Can I really do this on my own? I've tried. And tried. If God can create me so perfectly, then surely he can make my life right and show me my purpose.

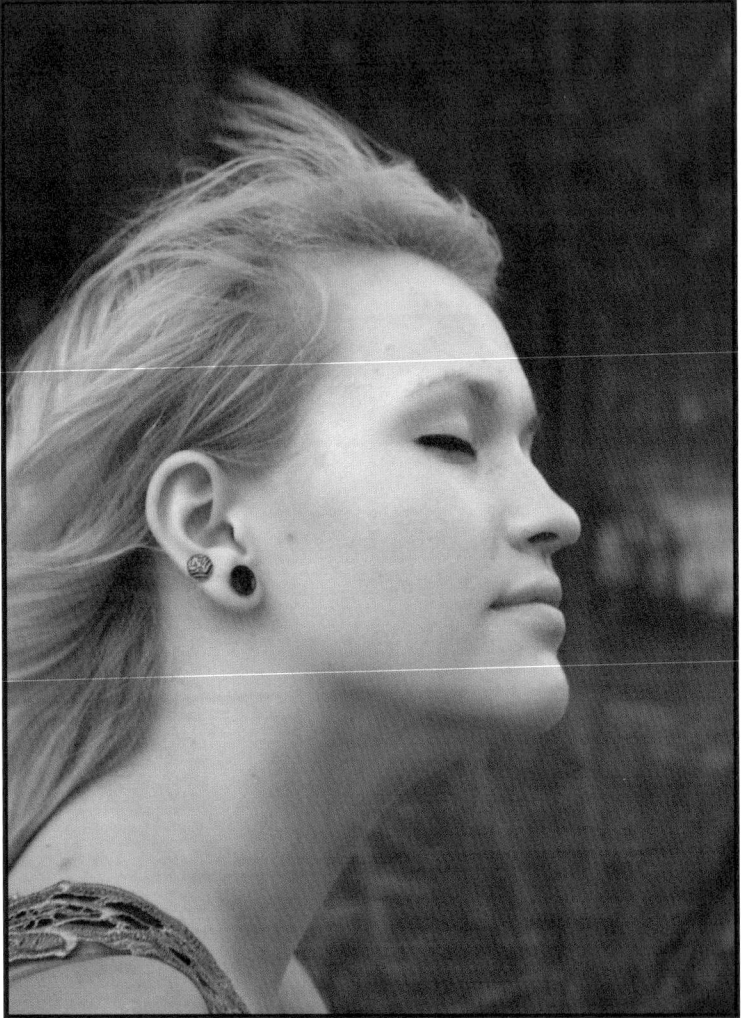

Someone told me once that if you ever wonder if God has a purpose for your life, check to see if you're breathing. If you are, then he does. I am. And that's another miracle. I mean, how do people breathe anyway, and who came up with that? Like oxygen and lungs and how the lungs work and everything. It's insane. Insanely perfect. God, of course.

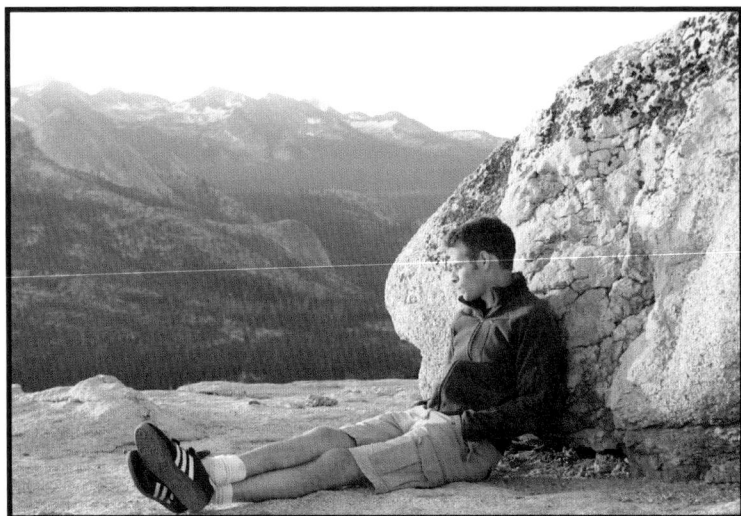

Why would he do all of that for me? For ME? Little old me, lying here existing, a ball of dust (but very special dust), who doesn't believe I can do anything.

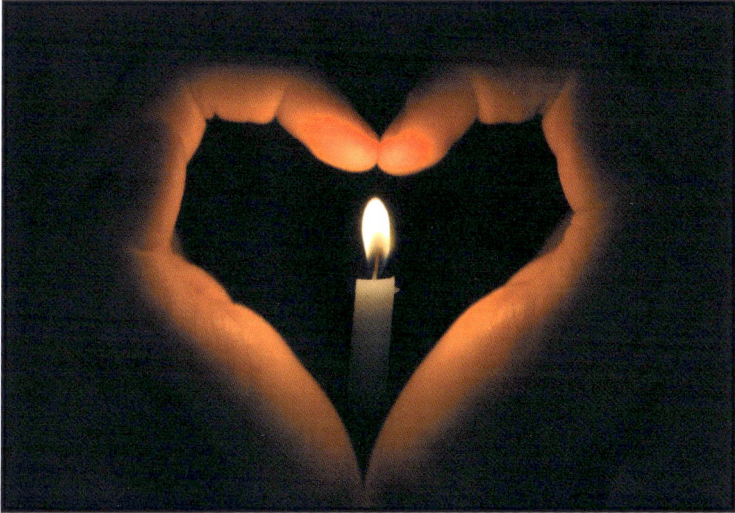

I know God is love. Is that the way he loves? Would he create something he doesn't love? And even if he did create something and it turned out to be so bad and vile that he didn't love it anymore, or that it didn't deserve love anymore, would he still keep my heart beating? Would he keep blood running through me?

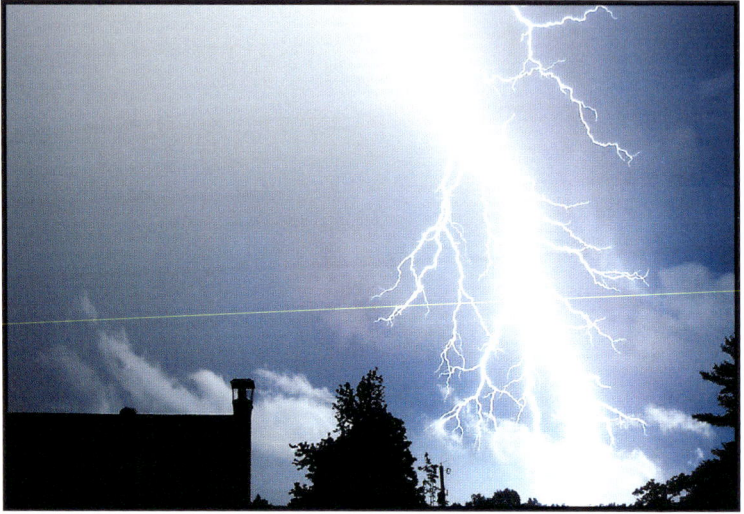

Wouldn't he just zap me out of existence and say "well, that one turned out to be no good." He could. Make me vanish, that is. If he can create me, he could certainly wipe me off this earth just as easily. So why hasn't he? Why am I still lying here existing?

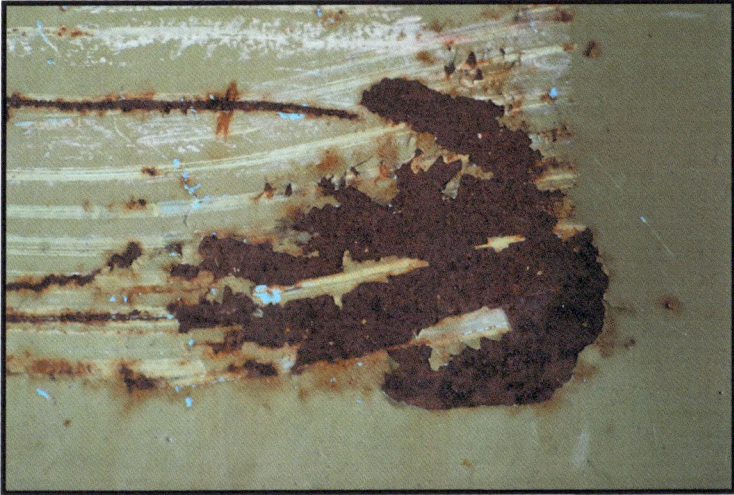

Maybe, for some reason, God thinks I deserve another chance. Maybe, underneath all the pain and the broken soul and the screwed up life and the scars he sees a different me. A better me. Maybe he sees what I COULD be instead of who I am right now. Maybe he sees what I WILL be instead of who I am right now. Wish I could see it.

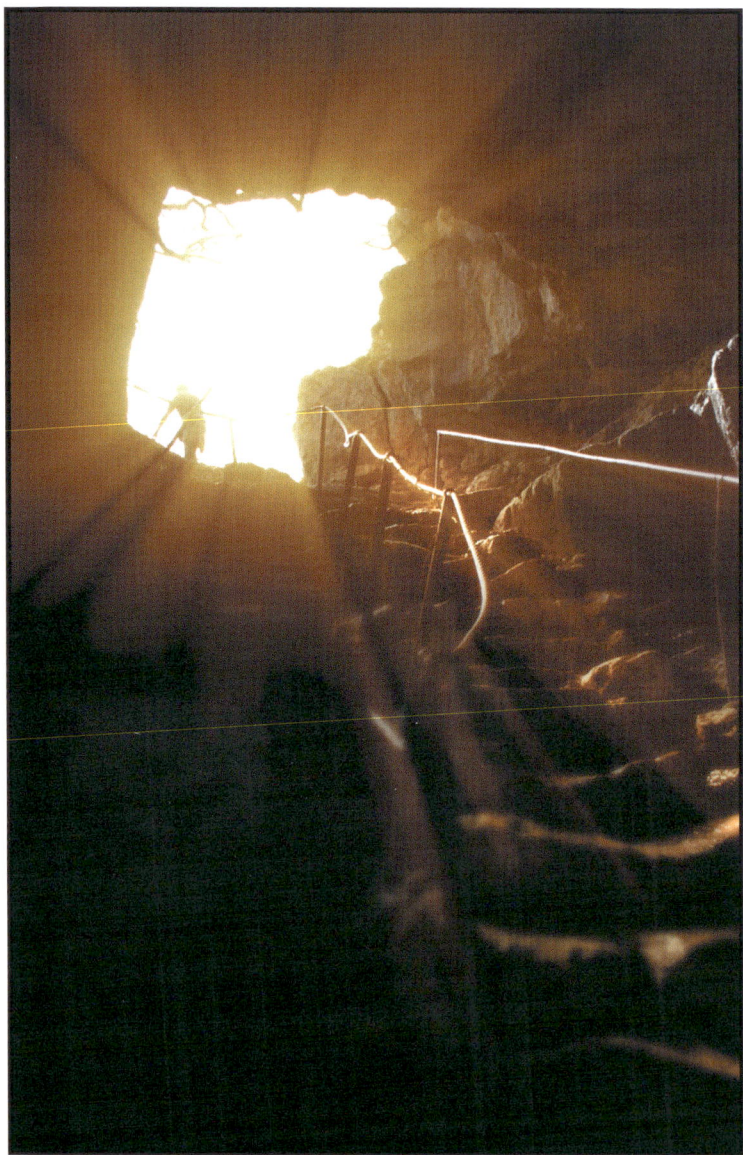

If he sees it, will he help me become that person?

The one that he thinks deserves to live?

Will he give me strength?

Will he give me hope?

He's gonna have to because I don't have any of my own right now.

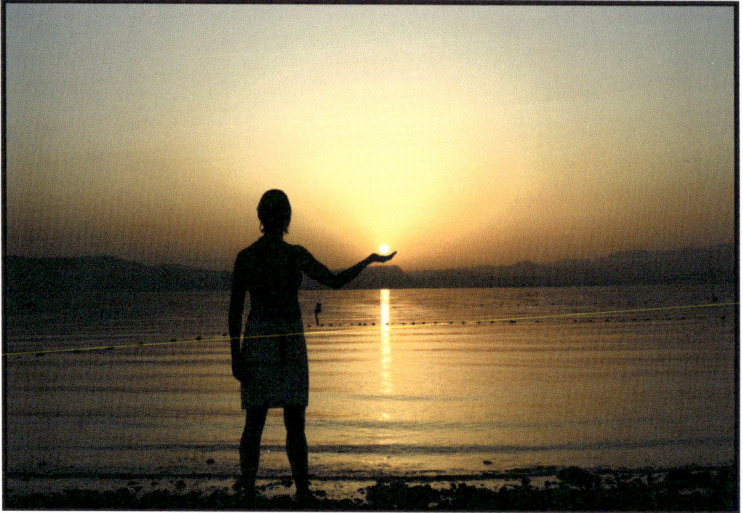

All I have is the fact that I am
still breathing so I must have
a purpose, my heart is still
beating because God touched it
and started it pumping, and I
was incredibly created by God,
different from everyone else, with
my own DNA. He didn't even give
that to the stars.

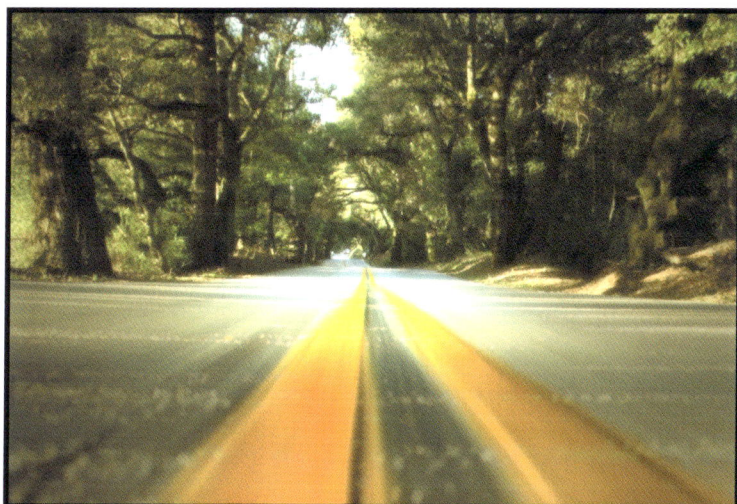

I am alive.

Even though my heart may not feel like it yet, I must have a chance, because God thinks I have a chance, and one day he will show me what that purpose is.

He has to, because I'm still breathing.

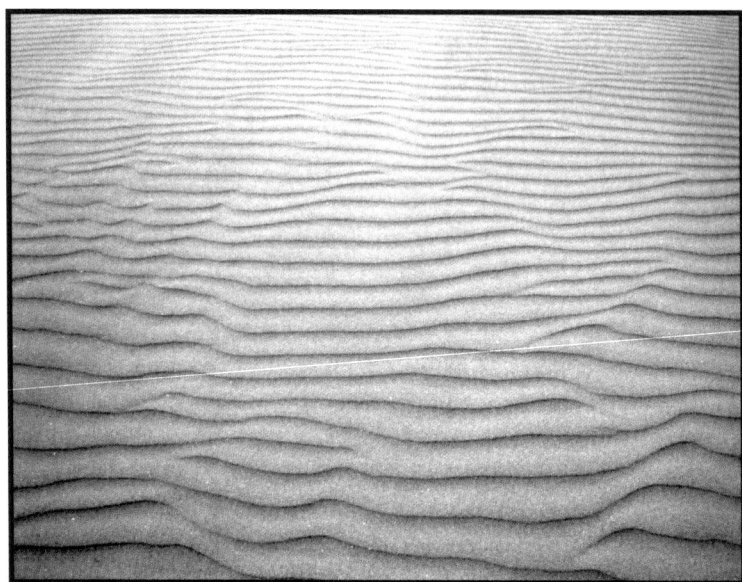

I am nothing. I am no one. I am
just a bunch of dust put together.
But I am God's nothing, and that
makes me something. And I am
God's no one, so that makes me
someone. I am just a bunch of
dust put together, but I am made
of very special dust that can do
things that no one else can do.

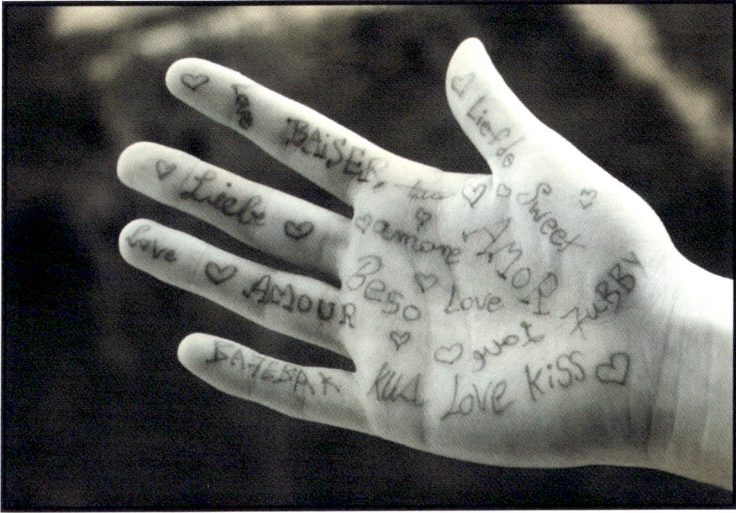

I am wonderfully made by God,
even better than the stars. I am
a miracle. I am God's very own
miracle made because of love. I
may not have much strength right
now, and it may take a while
to get it back. But I am God's
creation, and if he can create me,
he can give me strength.

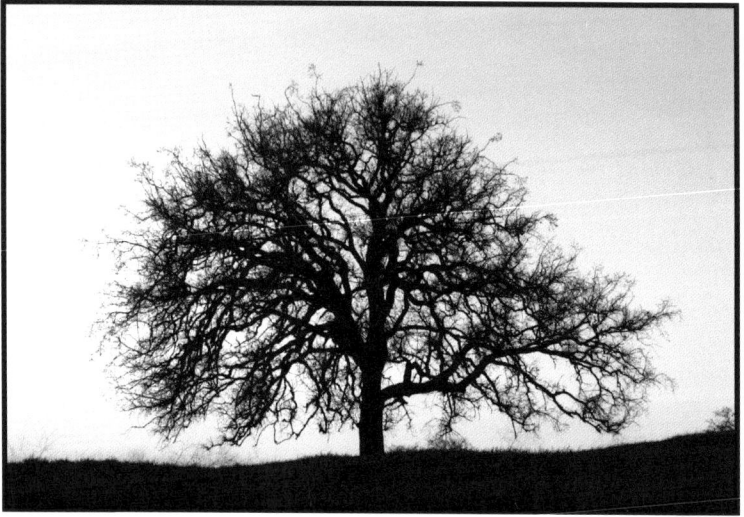

Strength...

in the middle...

of pain...

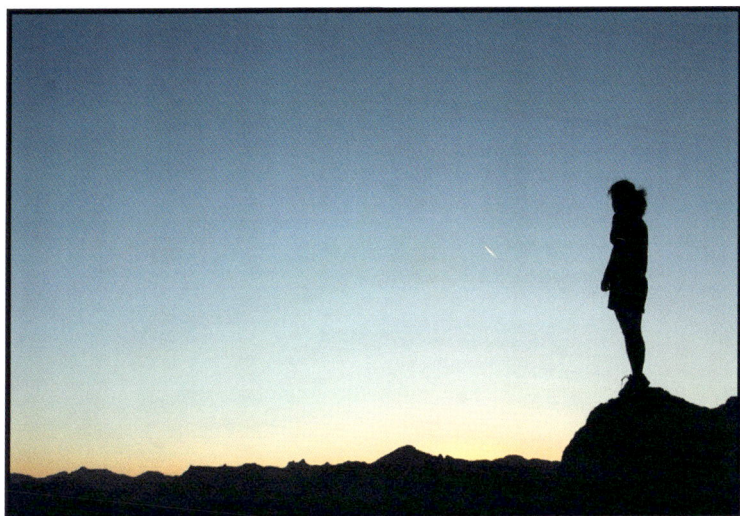

I am different. I am wonderful.

I am loved, even when it seems
like love is gone.

I am me.

And I am still breathing...

Information:

Suicide Hotline

1-800-273-TALK (8255)

www.suicidepreventionlifeline.org

Alcoholics Anonymous

(212) 870-3400

www.aa.org

Recovery for Drug or Alcohol Addiction (and more)

www.addictions.org

www.liferecoveryproducts.com

Find a Therapist

www.psychologytoday.com

www.goodtherapy.org

Info About Studying the Bible

www.newlivingtranslation.com

45

Credits:

Thank you to all the photographers who contributed their work to this project. Without you, this book would not exist.

Images on pages 4, 6, 11, 12, 16, 19, 33, 34 and 40 are by Sam Mugraby and are courtesy of Photos8.com

Images on pages 17, 21, 22, 25, 28, 32, 36, 37, 38, 39, 41 and 42 are by David Niblack and are courtesy of ImageBase. imagebase.davidniblack.com

Images on pages 10, 27, 29, 30, and 35 are by Alegri and are courtesy of 4FreePhotos.com

Image on page 18 is by McRaffael and is courtesy of 4FreePhotos.com

Images on pages 5, 7, 8, 14 and 15 are by NASA and are courtesy of NasaImages.org

Image on page 9 is by Magnus Rosendahl and is courtesy of FreePhotos.se

Image on page 13 is by Tinka Sloss for a NASA-funded project and is courtesy of Serc.Carleton.edu

Image on page 20 is by Liz Lawley and is courtesy of Commons. Wikimedia.org

Image on page 24 is by Francesco Marino and is courtesy of FreeDigitalPhotos.net

Image on page 31 is by Benjamin Miller and is courtesy of FreeStockPhotos.biz

Images on pages 23 and 26 are by Sherri Gough and are courtesy of Steel Train Publishing

Author Photo is by Anthony Scarlati

Permission is granted to use this material for discussion in 12-step programs or other therapy programs, when under the supervision of a licensed counselor or professional minister, and according to the terms of the contracts of the individual image owners.

47

Who am I?

I am not a counselor. I am not a teacher. I don't have my PhD in Psychology. I don't lead addiction-based recovery programs, or help people cope with depression.

You might be wondering what right I have to write this book.

I don't have any "right" to write this book, actually. I'm a songwriter, a performer, an author, a wife, a mom, and I have a degree in Economics, not Psychology. Oh yeah, and I am also a PERSON.

I've seen friends and acquaintances that I work with in the music industry struggle with issues of insecurity, hopelessness, addiction, depression, and worthlessness. Creative people have a greater tendency to feel more strongly and deeply, which leaves them more vulnerable to these issues.

I'm just a person who wants to let other people know that they are loved unconditionally, no matter what, scars and all, with all of their addictions and failures attached, by the God of the universe. And that's all. When this world doesn't love you and you don't even love yourself, God does. When you can hardly function and life is overwhelming and you feel invisible, he sees you.

Life goes in cycles, so when it's dark, let it be dark and just hold on. Wait for a new chapter to come around. Wait for healing to find you if you don't have the strength to reach for it.

I have been in good times and really brutal, heart-wrenching times of my life. I don't claim to know your struggles, but I do know that I have certainly learned a lot from mine.

There's no one with greater faith than the person who feels unworthy of God's love. If someone feels "worthy" and thinks they deserve his love because they're a pretty good person, how can they possibly know what GRACE is all about?

When we are humble and broken, only then can we start to fully rely on God...because we have to. If you are one of those broken people... congratulations. You have a head start above everyone else in realizing what true, unconditional love is all about.

If you don't know how to pray but want to, just tell God three words..."I'm not worthy." Keep telling him that. When you can't think of anything else to say, say that. Every day, tell God you're not worthy of his love, but you'll take it anyway. And, now look...you're praying. Now all you have to do is continue the conversation. ☺

I'm not an expert on life. I'm not an expert on God. I'm not an expert on psychology. I'm certainly not an expert on you and your own personal pain. But I'm an expert on being a person, because I am one. And you are too.

I hope that the ramblings of my heart in this book will give you some sort of light, some sort of purpose, and some sort of hope. And I hope you realize that no one else can ever be you.

Keep breathing...

Sherri

yourself, God does. When you can hardly function and life is overwhelming and you feel invisible, he sees you.

Life goes in cycles, so when it's dark, let it be dark and just hold on. Wait for a new chapter to come around. Wait for healing to find you if you don't have the strength to reach for it.

I have been in good times and really brutal, heart-wrenching times of my life. I don't claim to know your struggles, but I do know that I have certainly learned a lot from mine.

There's no one with greater faith than the person who feels unworthy of God's love. If someone feels "worthy" and thinks they deserve his love because they're a pretty good person, how can they possibly know what GRACE is all about?

When we are humble and broken, only then can we start to fully rely on God…because we have to. If you are one of those broken people… congratulations. You have a head start above everyone else in realizing what true, unconditional love is all about.

If you don't know how to pray but want to, just tell God three words…"I'm not worthy." Keep telling him that. When you can't think of anything else to say, say that. Every day, tell God you're not worthy of his love, but you'll take it anyway. And, now look...you're praying. Now all you have to do is continue the conversation. ☺

I'm not an expert on life. I'm not an expert on God. I'm not an expert on psychology. I'm certainly not an expert on you and your own personal pain. But I'm an expert on being a person, because I am one. And you are too.

I hope that the ramblings of my heart in this book will give you some sort of light, some sort of purpose, and some sort of hope. And I hope you realize that no one else can ever be you.

Keep breathing...

Sherri